# Best Guide to Keto Diet Recipes

*Best Guide with Delicious Ketogenic Recipes Low Carbs for Healthy Weight Loss*

Sarah Vellar

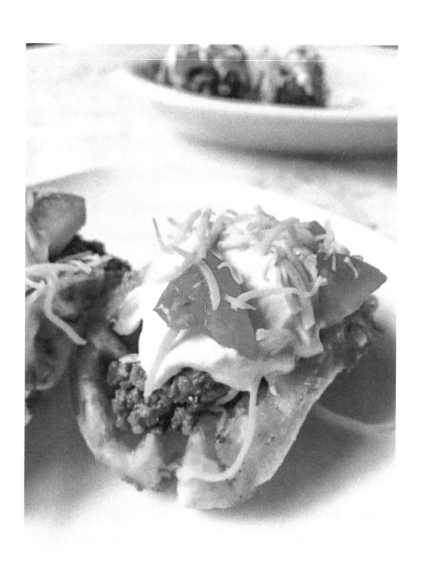

# Table of Contents

The information in the following pages is broadly considered a truthful and accurate account of facts and as such, any inattention, use, or misuse of the information in question by the reader will render any resulting actions solely under their purview. There are no scenarios in which the publisher or the original author of this work can be in any fashion deemed liable for any hardship or damages that may befall them after undertaking information described herein.

Additionally, the information in the following pages is intended only for informational purposes and should thus be thought of as universal. As befitting its nature, it is presented without assurance regarding its prolonged validity or interim quality. Trademarks that are mentioned are done without written consent and can in no way be considered an endorsement from the trademark holder.

# INTRODUCTION

So the Ketogenic Diet is all about reducing the amount of carbohydrates you eat. Does this mean you won't get the kind of energy you need for the day? Of course not! It only means that now, your body has to find other possible sources of energy. Do you know where they will be getting that energy? Even before we talk about how to do keto – it's important to first consider why this particular diet works. What actually happens to your body to make you lose weight? As you probably know, the body uses food as an energy source. Everything you eat is turned into energy, so that you can get up and do whatever you need to accomplish for the day. The main energy source is sugar so what happens is that you eat something, the body breaks it down into sugar, and the sugar is processed into energy. Typically, the "sugar" is taken directly from the food you eat so if you eat just the right amount of food, then your body is fueled for the whole day. If you eat too much, then the sugar is stored in your body – hence the accumulation of fat.

But what happens if you eat less food? This is where the Ketogenic Diet comes in. You see, the process of creating sugar from food is usually faster if the food happens to be rich in carbohydrates. Bread, rice, grain, pasta – all of these are carbohydrates and they're the easiest food types to turn into energy. So here's the situation – you are eating less carbohydrates every day. To keep you energetic, the body breaks down the stored fat and turns them into molecules called ketone bodies. The process of turning the fat into ketone bodies is called "Ketosis" and obviously – this is where the name of the Ketogenic Diet comes from. The ketone bodies take the place of glucose in keeping you energetic. As long as you keep your carbohydrates reduced, the body will keep getting its energy from your body fat. The Ketogenic Diet is often praised for its simplicity and when you look at it properly, the process is really straightforward. The Science behind the effectivity of the diet is also well-documented, and has been proven multiple times by different medical fields. For example, an article on Diet Review by Harvard provided a lengthy discussion on how the Ketogenic Diet works and why it is so effective for those who choose to use this diet. But Fat Is the Enemy...Or Is It? No – fat is NOT the enemy. Unfortunately, years of bad science told us that fat is something you have to avoid – but it's actually a very helpful thing for weight loss! Even before we move forward with this book, we'll have to discuss exactly what "healthy fats" are, and why they're actually the good guys. To do this, we need to make a distinction between the different kinds of fat. You've probably heard of them before and it is a little bit confusing at first. We'll try to go through them as simply as possible: Saturated fat. This is the kind you want to avoid. They're also called "solid fat" because each molecule is packed with hydrogen atoms. Simply put, it's the kind of fat that can easily cause a blockage in your body. It can raise cholesterol levels and lead to heart problems or a stroke. Saturated fat is something you can find in meat, dairy products, and other processed food items. Now, you're probably wondering: isn't the Ketogenic Diet packed with saturated fat? The answer is: not necessarily. You'll find later in the recipes given that the Ketogenic Diet promotes primarily unsaturated fat or healthy fat. While there are definitely many meat recipes in the list, most of these recipes contain healthy fat sources.

Unsaturated Fat. These are the ones dubbed as healthy fat. They're the kind of fat you find in avocado, nuts, and other ingredients you usually find in Keto-friendly recipes. They're known to lower blood cholesterol and actually come in two types: polyunsaturated and monounsaturated. Both are good for your body but the benefits slightly vary, depending on what you're consuming.

# Buffalo Chicken Sausage Balls

**Preparation Time: 5 minutes**

**Cooking Time: 25 minutes**

**Servings: 2**

**Ingredients:**

- Sausage Balls:
- 2 14-ox sausages, casings removed
- 2 cups almond flour
- 1 ½ cups shredded cheddar cheese
- ½ cup crumbled bleu cheese
- 1 tsp salt
- ½ tsp pepper
- Bleu Cheese Ranch Dipping Sauce:
- 1/3 cup mayonnaise
- 1/3 cup almond milk, unsweetened
- 2 cloves garlic, minced
- 1 tsp dried dill
- ½ tsp dried parsley
- ½ tsp salt
- ½ tsp pepper
- ¼ cup crumbled bleu cheese (or more, if desired)

## Directions:

1. Preheat your oven at 35o degrees F.

2. Layer two baking sheets with wax paper and set them aside.

3. Mix sausage with cheddar cheese, almond flour, salt, pepper, and bleu cheese in a large bowl.

4. Make 1-inch balls out of this mixture and place them on the baking sheets.

5. Bake them for 25 minutes until golden brown.

6. Meanwhile, prepare the dipping sauce by whisking all of its ingredients in a bowl.

7. Serve the balls with this dipping sauce.

**Nutrition:** Calories: 183 Fat: 15 g Cholesterol 11 mg Sodium 31 mg Total carbohydrates 6.2 g Protein 4.5 g

# Brussels Sprouts Chips

**Preparation Time: 5 minutes**

**Cooking Time: 15 minutes**

**Servings: 6**

**Ingredients:**

- 1-pound Brussels sprouts, washed and dried
- 2 tbsp. extra virgin olive oil
- 1 tsp kosher salt

**Directions:**

1. Preheat your oven at 400 degrees F.
2. After peeling the sprouts off the stem, discard the outer leaves of the Brussel sprouts.
3. Separate all the leaves from one another and place them on a baking sheet.
4. Toss them with oil and salt thoroughly to coat them well.
5. Spread the leaves out on two greased baking sheets then bake them for 15 minutes until crispy.
6. Serve.

**Nutrition:** Calories: 188 Fat: 3 g Cholesterol: 101

Sodium: 54 mg Fiber 0.6 g Protein 5 g

# Keto Chocolate Mousse

**Preparation Time: 5 minutes**

**Cooking Time: 0 minutes**

**Servings: 2**

**Ingredients:**

- 1 cup heavy whipping cream
- ¼ cup unsweetened cocoa powder, sifted
- ¼ cup Swerve powdered sweetener
- 1 tsp vanilla extract
- ¼ tsp kosher salt

**Directions:**

1. Add cream to the bowl of an electric stand mixture and beat it until it forms peaks.
2. Stir in cocoa powder, vanilla, sweetener, and salt.
3. Mix well until smooth.
4. Refrigerate for 4 hours.
5. Serve.

**Nutrition:** Calories: 153 Fat: 13 g Cholesterol: 6.5 mg Sodium: 81 mg Sugar 1.4 g Protein 5.8 g

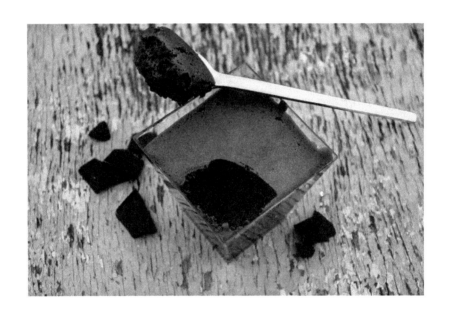

# Keto Berry Mousse

**Preparation Time: 5 minutes**

**Cooking Time: 0 minutes**

**Servings: 2**

**Ingredients:**

- 2 cups heavy whipping cream
- 3 oz. fresh raspberries
- 2 oz. chopped pecans
- ½ lemon, zested
- ¼ tsp vanilla extract

**Directions:**

1. Beat cream in a bowl using a hand mixer until it forms peaks.
2. Stir in vanilla and lemon zest and mix well until incorporated.
3. Fold in nuts and berries and mix well.
4. Cover the mixture with plastic wrap and refrigerate for 3 hours.
5. Serve fresh.

**Nutrition:** Calories: 254 Fat: 9 g Cholesterol: 13 mg Sodium: 179 mg Sugar 1.2 g Protein 7.5 g

# Peanut Butter Mousse

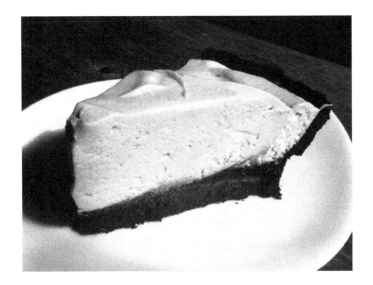

**Preparation Time: 5 minutes**

**Cooking Time: 0 minutes**

**Servings: 4**

**Ingredients:**

- ½ cup heavy whipping cream
- 4 oz. cream cheese, softened
- ¼ cup natural peanut butter
- ¼ cup powdered Swerve sweetener
- ½ tsp vanilla extract

**Direction:**

1. Beat ½ cup cream in a medium bowl with a hand mixer until it forms peaks.
2. Beat cream cheese with peanut butter in another bowl until creamy.
3. Stir in vanilla, a pinch of salt, and sweetener to the peanut butter mix and combine until smooth.
4. Fold in the prepared whipped cream and mix well until fully incorporated.
5. Divide the mousse into 4 serving glasses.
6. Garnish as desired.
7. Enjoy.

**Nutrition:** Calories: 290 Fat: 21.5 Cholesterol: 12 Sodium: 9 Protein: 6

# Cookie Ice Cream

**Preparation Time: 10 minutes**

**Cooking Time: 120 minutes**

**Servings: 2**

**Ingredients:**

- Cookie Crumbs
- ¾ cup almond flour
- ¼ cup cocoa powder
- ¼ tsp baking soda
- ¼ cup erythritol
- ½ tsp vanilla extract
- 1 ½ tbsp. coconut oil, softened
- 1 large egg, room temperature
- Pinch of salt
- Ice Cream
- 2 ½ cups whipping cream
- 1 tbsp. vanilla extract
- ½ cup erythritol
- ½ cup almond milk, unsweetened

**Directions:**

1. Preheat your oven at 300 degrees F and layer a 9-inch baking pan with wax paper.
2. Whisk almond flour with baking soda, cocoa powder, salt, and erythritol in a medium bowl.
3. Stir in coconut oil and vanilla extract then mix well until crumbly.
4. Whisk in egg and mix well to form the dough.
5. Spread this dough in the prepared pan and bake for 20 minutes in the preheated oven.
6. Allow the crust to cool then crush it finely into crumbles.
7. Beat cream in a large bowl with a hand mixer until it forms a stiff peak.
8. Stir in erythritol and vanilla extract then mix well until fully incorporated.
9. Pour in milk and blend well until smooth.
10. Add this mixture to an ice cream machine and churn as per the machine's instructions.
11. Add cookie crumbles to the ice cream in the machine and churn again.
12. Place the ice cream in a sealable container and freeze for 2 hours.
13. Scoop out the ice cream and serve.

14. Enjoy.

15. *Note:* this recipe calls for an ice cream machine

**Nutrition:** Calories: 214 Fat: 19 Cholesterol: 15 Sodium: 12 Fiber: 2 Protein: 7

# Mocha Ice Cream

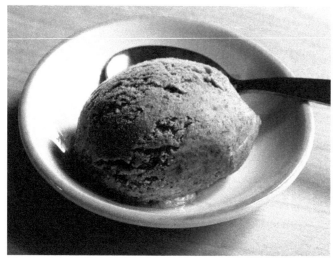

**Preparation Time: 10 minutes**

**Cooking Time: 0 minutes**

**Servings: 2**

**Ingredients:**

- 1 cup coconut milk

- ¼ cup heavy whipping cream

- 2 tbsp. erythritol

- 15 drops liquid stevia

- 2 tbsp. unsweetened cocoa powder

- 1 tbsp. instant coffee

- ¼ tsp xanthan gum

**Directions:**

1. Whisk everything except xanthan gum in a bowl using a hand mixer.
2. Slowly add xanthan gum and stir well to make a thick mixture.
3. Churn the mixture in an ice cream machine as per the machine's instructions.
4. Freeze it for 2 hours then garnish with mint and instant coffee.
5. Serve.
6. *Note:* this recipe calls for an ice cream machine

**Nutrition:** Calories: 267 Fat: 44.5 g Cholesterol: 153 mg Sodium: 217 mg

# Raspberry Cream Fat Bombs

**Preparation Time: 10 minutes**

**Cooking Time: 0 minutes**

**Servings: 2**

**Ingredients:**

- 1 packet raspberry Jello (sugar-free)
- 1 tsp gelatin powder
- ½ cup of boiling water
- ½ cup heavy cream

**Directions:**

1. Mix Jello and gelatin in boiling water in a medium bowl.
2. Stir in cream slowly and mix it for 1 minute.
3. Divide this mixture into candy molds.
4. Refrigerate them for 30 minutes.
5. Enjoy.

**Nutrition:** Calories: 197 Fat: 19.2 g Cholesterol: 11 mg Sodium: 78 mg

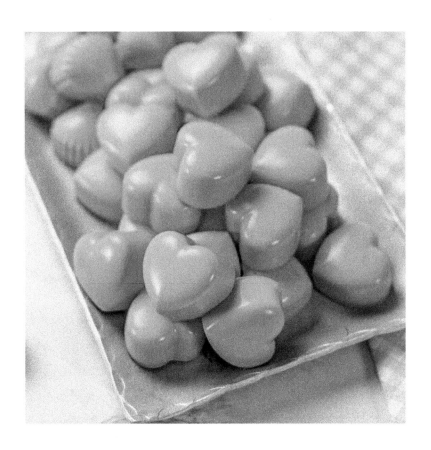

# Cauliflower Tartar Bread

**Preparation Time: 10 minutes**

**Cooking Time: 50 minutes**

**Servings: 4**

**Ingredients:**

- 3 cup cauliflower rice
- 10 large eggs, yolks and egg whites separated
- ¼ tsp cream of tartar
- 1 ¼ cup coconut flour
- 1 ½ tbsp. gluten-free baking powder
- 1 tsp sea salt
- 6 tbsp. butter
- 6 cloves garlic, minced
- 1 tbsp. fresh rosemary, chopped
- 1 tbsp. fresh parsley, chopped

**Directions:**

1. Preheat your oven to 350 degrees F. Layer a 9x5-inch pan with wax paper.
2. Place the cauliflower rice in a suitable bowl and then cover it with plastic wrap.

3. Heat it for 4 minutes in the microwave. Heat more if the cauliflower isn't soft enough.
4. Place the cauliflower rice in a kitchen towel and squeeze it to drain excess water.
5. Transfer drained cauliflower rice to a food processor.
6. Add coconut flour, sea salt, baking powder, butter, egg yolks, and garlic. Blend until crumbly.
7. Beat egg whites with cream of tartar in a bowl until foamy.
8. Add egg white mixture to the cauliflower mixture and stir well with a spatula.
9. Fold in rosemary and parsley.
10. Spread this batter in the prepared baking pan evenly.
11. Bake it for 50 minutes until golden then allow it to cool.

**Nutrition:** Calories: 104 Fat: 8.9 g Cholesterol: 57 mg Sodium: 340 mg Carbohydrates: 4.7 g

# Buttery Skillet Flatbread

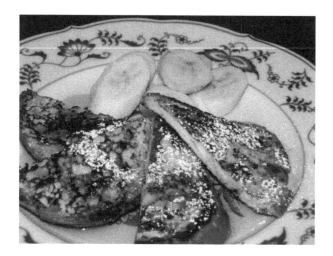

**Preparation Time: 10 minutes**

**Cooking Time: 10 minutes**

**Servings: 4**

**Ingredients:**

- 1 cup almond flour
- 2 tbsp. coconut flour
- 2 tsp xanthan gum
- ½ tsp baking powder
- ½ tsp salt
- 1 whole egg + 1 egg white
- 1 tbsp. water (if needed)
- 1 tbsp. oil, for frying

- 1 tbsp. melted butter, for brushing

## Directions:

1. Mix xanthan gum with flours, salt, and baking powder in a suitable bowl.

2. Beat egg and egg white in a separate bowl then stir in the flour mixture.

3. Mix well until smooth. Add a tablespoon of water if the dough is too thick.

4. Place a large skillet over medium heat and heat oil.

**Nutrition:** Calories: 272 Fat: 18 Cholesterol: 6.1

# Fluffy Bites

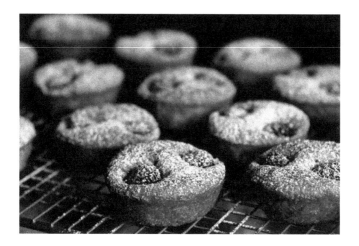

**Preparation Time: 20 minutes**

**Cooking Time: 60 minutes**

**Servings: 12**

**Ingredients:**

- 2 Teaspoons Cinnamon
- 2/3 Cup Sour Cream
- 2 Cups Heavy Cream
- 1 Teaspoon Scraped Vanilla Bean
- ¼ Teaspoon Cardamom
- 4 Egg Yolks
- Stevia to Taste

**Directions:**

1. Start by whisking your egg yolks until creamy and smooth.

2. Get out a double boiler, and add your eggs with the rest of your ingredients. Mix well.

3. Remove from heat, allowing it to cool until it reaches room temperature.

4. Refrigerate for an hour before whisking well.

5. Pour into molds, and freeze for at least an hour before serving.

**Nutrition:** Calories: 363 Protein: 2 Fat: 40 Carbohydrates: 1

# Coconut Fudge

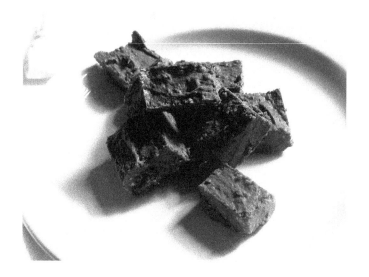

**Preparation Time: 20 minutes**

**Cooking Time: 60 minutes**

**Servings: 12**

**Ingredients:**

- 2 Cups Coconut Oil
- ½ Cup Dark Cocoa Powder
- ½ Cup Coconut Cream
- ¼ Cup Almonds, Chopped
- ¼ Cup Coconut, Shredded
- 1 Teaspoon Almond Extract
- Pinch of Salt

- Stevia to Taste

## Directions:

1. Pour your coconut oil and coconut cream in a bowl, whisking with an electric beater until smooth. Once the mixture becomes smooth and glossy, do not continue.

2. Begin to add in your cocoa powder while mixing slowly, making sure that there aren't any lumps.

3. Add in the rest of your ingredients, and mix well.

4. Line a bread pan with parchment paper, and freeze until it sets.

5. Slice into squares before serving.

**Nutrition:** Calories: 172 Fat: 20 Carbohydrates: 3

# Nutmeg Nougat

**Preparation Time: 30 minutes**

**Cooking Time: 60 minutes**

**Servings: 12**

**Ingredients:**

- 1 Cup Heavy Cream
- 1 Cup Cashew Butter
- 1 Cup Coconut, Shredded
- ½ Teaspoon Nutmeg
- 1 Teaspoon Vanilla Extract, Pure
- Stevia to Taste

**Directions:**

1. Melt your cashew butter using a double boiler, and then stir in your vanilla extract, dairy cream, nutmeg and stevia. Make sure it's mixed well.
2. Remove from heat, allowing it to cooldown before refrigerating it for a half hour.
3. Shape into balls, and coat with shredded coconut. Chill for at least two hours before serving.

**Nutrition:** Calories: 341 Fat: 34 Carbohydrates: 5

# Sweet Almond Bites

**Preparation Time: 30 minutes**

**Cooking Time: 90 minutes**

**Servings: 12**

**Ingredients:**

- 18 Ounces Butter, Grass Fed
- 2 Ounces Heavy Cream
- ½ Cup Stevia
- 2/3 Cup Cocoa Powder
- 1 Teaspoon Vanilla Extract, Pure
- 4 Tablespoons Almond Butter

**Direction:**

1. Use a double boiler to melt your butter before adding in all of your remaining ingredients.
2. Place the mixture into molds, freezing for two hours before serving.

**Nutrition:** Calories: 350 Protein: 2 Fat: 38

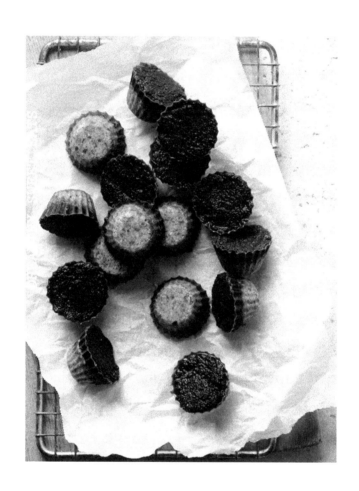

# Strawberry Cheesecake Minis

**Preparation Time: 30 minutes**

**Cooking Time: 120 minutes**

**Servings: 12**

**Ingredients:**

- 1 Cup Coconut Oil
- 1 Cup Coconut Butter
- ½ Cup Strawberries, Sliced
- ½ Teaspoon Lime Juice
- 2 Tablespoons Cream Cheese, Full Fat
- Stevia to Taste

**Directions:**

1. Blend your strawberries together.
2. Soften your cream cheese, and then add in your coconut butter.
3. Combine all ingredients together, and then pour your mixture into silicone molds.
4. Freeze for at least two hours before serving.

**Nutrition:** Calories: 372 Protein: 1 Fat: 41 Carbohydrates: 2

# Cocoa Brownies

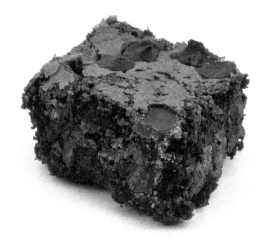

**Preparation Time: 10 minutes**

**Cooking Time: 30 minutes**

**Servings: 12**

**Ingredients:**

- 1 Egg
- 2 Tablespoons Butter, Grass Fed
- 2 Teaspoons Vanilla Extract, Pure
- ¼ Teaspoon Baking Powder
- ¼ Cup Cocoa Powder
- 1/3 Cup Heavy Cream
- ¾ Cup Almond Butter

- Pinch Sea Salt

## Directions:

1. Break your egg into a bowl, whisking until smooth.
2. Add in all of your wet ingredients, mixing well.
3. Mix all dry ingredients into a bowl.
4. Sift your dry ingredients into your wet ingredients, mixing to form a batter.
5. Get out a baking pan, greasing it before pouring in your mixture.
6. Heat your oven to 350 and bake for twenty-five minutes.
7. Allow it to cool before slicing and serve room temperature or warm.

**Nutrition:** Calories: 184 Protein: 1 Fat: 20 Carbohydrates: 1

# Chocolate Orange Bites

**Preparation Time: 20 minutes**

**Cooking Time: 120 minutes**

**Servings: 6**

**Ingredients:**

- 10 Ounces Coconut Oil
- 4 Tablespoons Cocoa Powder
- ¼ Teaspoon Blood Orange Extract
- Stevia to Taste

**Directions:**

1. Melt half of your coconut oil using a double boiler, and then add in your stevia and orange extract.

2. Get out candy molds, pouring the mixture into it. Fill each mold halfway, and then place in the fridge until they set.

3. Melt the other half of your coconut oil, stirring in your cocoa powder and stevia, making sure that the mixture is smooth with no lumps.

4. Pour into your molds, filling them up all the way, and then allow it to set in the fridge before serving.

**Nutrition:** Calories: 188 Protein: 1 Fat: 21

Carbohydrates: 5

# Caramel Cones

**Preparation Time: 25 minutes**

**Cooking Time: 120 minutes**

**Servings: 6**

**Ingredients:**

- 2 Tablespoons Heavy Whipping Cream
- 2 Tablespoons Sour Cream
- 1 Tablespoon Caramel Sugar
- 1 Teaspoon Sea Salt, Fine
- 1/3 Cup Butter, Grass Fed
- 1/3 Cup Coconut Oil
- Stevia to Taste

**Directions:**

1. Soften your coconut oil and butter, mixing together.
2. Mix all ingredients together to form a batter, and ten place them in molds.
3. Top with a little salt, and keep refrigerated until serving.

**Nutrition:** Calories: 100 Fat: 12 Grams Carbohydrates: 1

# Cinnamon Bites

**Preparation Time: 20 minutes**

**Cooking Time: 95 minutes**

**Servings: 6**

**Ingredients:**

- 1/8 Teaspoon Nutmeg
- 1 Teaspoon Vanilla Extract
- ¼ Teaspoon Cinnamon
- 4 Tablespoons Coconut Oil
- ½ Cup Butter, Grass Fed
- 8 Ounces Cream Cheese
- Stevia to Taste

**Directions:**

1. Soften your coconut oil and butter, mixing in your cream cheese.
2. Add all of your remaining ingredients, and mix well.
3. Pour into molds, and freeze until set.

**Nutrition:** Calories: 178 Protein: 1 Fat: 19

# Sweet Chai Bites

**Preparation Time: 20 minutes**

**Cooking Time: 45 minutes**

**Servings: 6**

**Ingredients:**

- 1 Cup Cream Cheese
- 1 Cup Coconut Oil
- 2 Ounces Butter, Grass Fed
- 2 Teaspoons Ginger
- 2 Teaspoons Cardamom
- 1 Teaspoon Nutmeg
- 1 Teaspoon Cloves
- 1 Teaspoon Vanilla Extract, Pure
- 1 Teaspoon Darjeeling Black Tea
- Stevia to Taste

**Directions:**

1. Melt your coconut oil and butter before adding in your black tea. Allow it to set for one to two minutes.
2. Add in your cream cheese, removing your mixture from heat.

3. Add in all of your spices, and stir to combine.

4. Pour into molds, and freeze before serving.

**Nutrition:** Calories: 178 Protein: 1 *Fat:* 19

# Easy Vanilla Bombs

**Preparation Time: 20 minutes**

**Cooking Time: 45 minutes**

**Servings: 14**

**Ingredients:**

- 1 Cup Macadamia Nuts, Unsalted
- ¼ Cup Coconut Oil / ¼ Cup Butter
- 2 Teaspoons Vanilla Extract, Sugar Free
- 20 Drops Liquid Stevia
- 2 Tablespoons Erythritol, Powdered

**Directions:**

1. Pulse your macadamia nuts in a blender, and then combine all of your ingredients together. Mix well.
2. Get out mini muffin tins with a tablespoon and a half of the mixture.
3. Refrigerate it for a half hour before serving.

**Nutrition:** Calories: 125 Fat: 5 Carbohydrates: 5

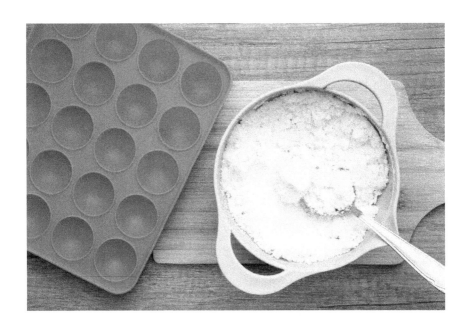

# Marinated Eggs

**Preparation Time: 2 hours and 10 minutes**

**Cooking Time: 7 minutes**

**Servings: 4**

**Ingredients:**

- 6 eggs
- 1 and ¼ cups water
- ¼ cup unsweetened rice vinegar 2 tablespoons coconut aminos
- Salt and black pepper to the taste 2 garlic cloves, minced
- 1 teaspoon stevia 4 ounces cream cheese
- 1 tablespoon chives, chopped

**Directions:**

1. Put the eggs in a pot, add water to cover, bring to a boil over medium heat, cover and cook for 7 minutes.
2. Rinse eggs with cold water and leave them aside to cool down.
3. In a bowl, mix 1 cup water with coconut aminos, vinegar, stevia and garlic and whisk well.

4. Put the eggs in this mix, cover with a kitchen towel and leave them aside for 2 hours rotating from time to time.

5. Peel eggs, cut in halves and put egg yolks in a bowl.

6. Add ¼ cup water, cream cheese, salt, pepper and chives and stir well.

7. Stuff egg whites with this mix and serve them.

8. Enjoy!

**Nutrition:** Calories: 289 kcal Protein: 15.86 g Fat: 22.62 g Carbohydrates: 4.52 g Sodium: 288 mg

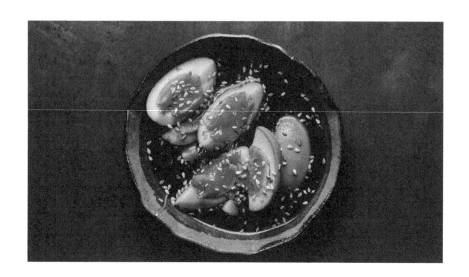

# Sausage and Cheese Dip

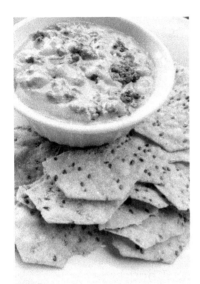

**Preparation Time: 10 minutes**

**Cooking Time: 130 minutes**

**Servings: 28**

**Ingredients:**

- 8 ounces cream cheese
- A pinch of salt and black pepper
- 16 ounces sour cream
- 8 ounces pepper jack cheese, chopped
- 15 ounces canned tomatoes mixed with habaneros
- 1 pound Italian sausage, ground
- ¼ cup green onions, chopped

## Directions:

1. Heat up a pan over medium heat, add sausage, stir and cook until it browns.
2. Add tomatoes mix, stir and cook for 4 minutes more.
3. Add a pinch of salt, pepper and the green onions, stir and cook for 4 minutes.
4. Spread pepper jack cheese on the bottom of your slow cooker.
5. Add cream cheese, sausage mix and sour cream, cover and cook on High for 2 hours.
6. Uncover your slow cooker, stir dip, transfer to a bowl and serve.
7. Enjoy!

**Nutrition:** Calories: 132 kcal Protein: 6.79 g Fat: 9.58 g Carbohydrates: 6.22 g Sodium: 362 mg

# Tasty Onion and Cauliflower Dip.

**Preparation Time: 20 minutes**

**Cooking Time: 30 minutes**

**Servings: 24**

**Ingredients:**

- 1 and ½ cups chicken stock
- 1 cauliflower head, florets separated
- ¼ cup mayonnaise
- ½ cup yellow onion, chopped
- ¾ cup cream cheese
- ½ teaspoon chili powder
- ½ teaspoon cumin, ground
- ½ teaspoon garlic powder
- Salt and black pepper to the taste

**Directions:**

1. Put the stock in a pot, add cauliflower and onion, heat up over medium heat and cook for 30 minutes.
2. Add chili powder, salt, pepper, cumin and garlic powder and stir.
3. Also add cream cheese and stir a bit until it melts.

4. Blend using an immersion blender and mix with the mayo.

5. Transfer to a bowl and keep in the fridge for 2 hours before you serve it.

6. Enjoy!

**Nutrition:** Calories: 40 kcal Protein: 1.23 g Fat: 3.31 g Carbohydrates: 1.66 g Sodium: 72 mg

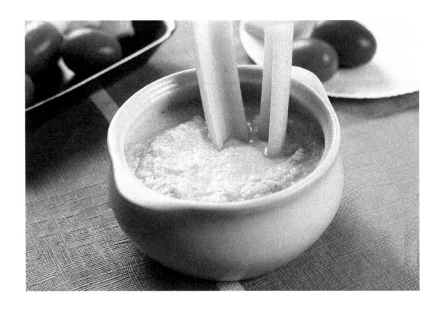

# Pesto Crackers

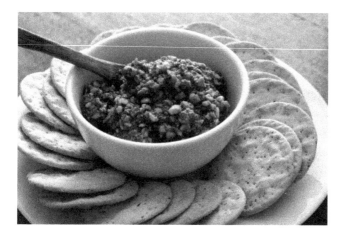

**Preparation Time: 10 minutes**

**Cooking Time: 17 minutes**

**Servings: 6**

**Ingredients**

- ½ teaspoon baking powder
- Salt and black pepper to the taste
- 1 and ¼ cups almond flour ¼ teaspoon basil, dried 1 garlic clove, minced
- 2 tablespoons basil pesto
- A pinch of cayenne pepper
- 3 tablespoons ghee

**Directions:**

1. In a bowl, mix salt, pepper, baking powder and almond flour.
2. Add garlic, cayenne and basil and stir.
3. Add pesto and whisk.
4. Also add ghee and mix your dough with your finger.
5. Spread this dough on a lined baking sheet, introduce in the oven at 325 degrees F and bake for 17 minutes.
6. Leave aside to cool down, cut your crackers and serve them as a snack.
7. Enjoy!

**Nutrition:** Calories: 9 kcal Protein: 0.41 g Fat: 0.14 g Carbohydrates: 1.86 g Sodium: 2 mg

# Pumpkin Muffins

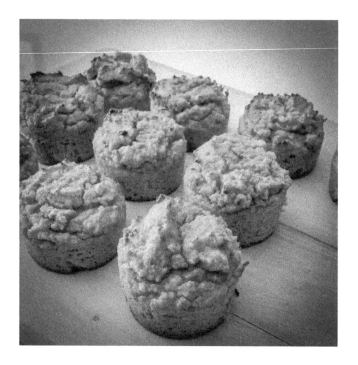

**Preparation Time: 10 minutes**

**Cooking Time: 15 minutes**

**Servings: 18**

**Ingredients:**

- ¼ cup sunflower seed butter
- ¾ cup pumpkin puree 2 tablespoons flaxseed meal ¼ cup coconut flour
- ½ cup erythritol ½ teaspoon nutmeg, ground

- 1 teaspoon cinnamon, ground ½ teaspoon baking soda 1 egg ½ teaspoon baking powder
- A pinch of salt

## Directions:

1. In a bowl, mix butter with pumpkin puree and egg and blend well.
2. Add flaxseed meal, coconut flour, erythritol, baking soda, baking powder, nutmeg, cinnamon and a pinch of salt and stir well.
3. Spoon this into a greased muffin pan, introduce in the oven at 350 degrees F and bake for 15 minutes.
4. Leave muffins to cool down and serve them as a snack.
5. Enjoy!

**Nutrition:** Calories: 65 kcal Protein: 2.82 g Fat: 5.42 g Carbohydrates: 2.27 g Sodium: 57 mg

# Keto Cornbread

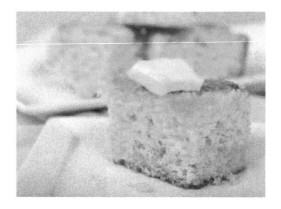

**Preparation Time**: 5 minutes;

**Cooking Time**: 2 minutes

**Servings**: 2

**Ingredients**

- 1 ¾ oz. almond flour
- ¼ tsp baking powder
- 1/8 tsp salt
- 1 tbsp. melted butter
- 1 egg

**Directions:**

1. Take a small bowl, place butter and egg in it, whisk until combined and then whisk in flour,

baking powder, and salt until smooth batter comes together.

2. Take a small microwave proof container, spoon prepared batter in it, and then microwave for 1 minute and 45 seconds at high heat setting until cooked.

3. When done, cut bread into slices, then spread with butter and serve.

**Nutrition**: 116.2 Calories; 10.4 g Fats; 4.3 g Protein; 1.1 g Net Carb; 1.5 g Fiber;

# Flax Seed Bread Sandwich

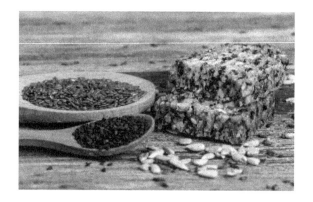

**Preparation Time**: 10 minutes

**Cooking Time**: 10 minutes

**Servings**: 2

**Ingredients**

- 4 oz. ground flaxseed
- 2 tsp coconut flour
- ½ tsp baking soda
- 1 tsp apple cider vinegar
- 2 tbsp. almond milk, unsweetened
- Seasoning:
- ¼ tsp sesame seeds
- ¼ tsp pumpkin seeds
- ¼ tsp sunflower seeds

- Peanut butter for serving

## Directions:

1. Take a medium bowl, place flaxseed in it, add flour, baking soda, vinegar, and milk and mix by using hand until smooth dough ball comes together.

2. Take a shallow dish, place sesame seeds, pumpkin seeds and sunflower seeds in it and then stir until mixed.

3. Divide dough ball into two pieces, roll each piece into a loaf and then press into seed mixture until evenly coated on both sides.

4. Place dough onto a heatproof plate, microwave for 1 minute and then cool breads for 5 minutes.

5. Slice each bread into half, then spread with peanut butter and serve.

**Nutrition**: 191 Calories; 15.1 g Fats; 4.8 g Protein; 1.2 g Net Carb; 7.1 g Fiber

# Cheesy Jalapeno Cornbread

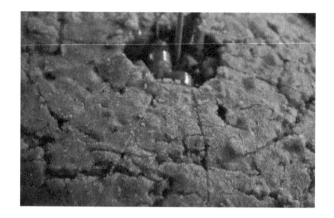

**Preparation Time**: 5 minutes;

**Cooking Time**: 2 minutes

**Servings**: 2

## Ingredients

- 1 jalapeno pepper, chopped
- 1 ¾ oz. almond flour
- ¼ tsp baking powder
- 1 egg
- 1 tbsp. grated parmesan cheese
- Seasoning:
- 1 tbsp. melted butter
- 1/8 tsp salt
- 1/8 tsp ground black pepper

## Directions:

1. Take a small bowl, place butter and egg in it, whisk until combined, and then whisk in remaining ingredients until smooth batter comes together.

2. Take a small microwave proof container, spoon prepared batter in it, and then microwave for 1 minute and 45 seconds at high heat setting until cooked.

3. When done, cut bread into slices, then spread with butter and serve.

**Nutrition**: 131 Calories; 11.1 g Fats; 4.8 g Protein; 1.1 g Net Carb; 0.9 g Fiber;

# Cheese Cup

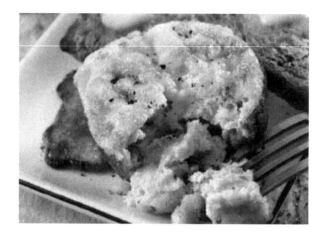

**Preparation Time**: 5 minutes

**Cooking Time**: 5 minutes

**Servings**: 2

**Ingredients**

- 4 tsp coconut flour
- 1/16 tsp baking soda
- 1 tbsp. grated mozzarella cheese
- 1 tbsp. grated parmesan cheese
- 2 eggs
- Seasoning:
- ¼ tsp salt
- ½ tsp dried basil

- ½ tsp dried parsley

## Directions:

1. Take a medium bowl, place all the ingredients in it, and whisk until well combined.

2. Take two ramekins, grease them with oil, distribute the prepared batter in it and then microwave for 1 minute and 45 seconds until done.

3. When done, take out muffin from the ramekin, cut in half, and then serve.

**Nutrition**: 125 Calories; 8.1 g Fats; 9.5 g Protein; 1.1 g Net Carb; 1.7 g Fiber;

# Cinnamon Mug Cake

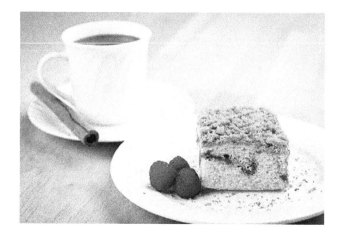

**Preparation Time**: 5 minutes;

**Cooking Time**: 5 minutes

**Servings**: 2

**Ingredients**

- 3 tbsp. almond flour
- 1 tbsp. erythritol sweetener
- 3 tbsp. butter, unsalted
- 2 tbsp. cream cheese
- 1 egg
- Seasoning:
- 1 tsp baking soda

- ¾ tsp cinnamon

## Directions:

1. Take a heatproof mug, place 2 tbsp. butter in it, and then microwave for 30 seconds or more until butter melts.
2. Then add remaining ingredients, reserving cream cheese and remaining butter, stir until mixed and microwave for 1 minute and 20 seconds until done.
3. Run a knife along the side of the mug and then take out the cake.
4. Melt the remaining butter, top it over the cake, then top with cream cheese, cut cake in half, and serve.

**Nutrition**: 298 Calories; 28.8 g Fats; 6.7 g Protein; 1.3 g Net Carb; 1.7 g Fiber;

# Spicy Dosa

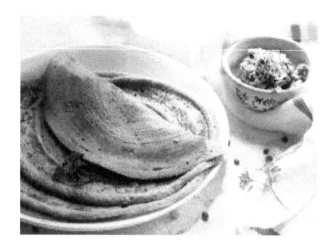

**Preparation Time**: 5 minutes;

**Cooking Time**: 8 minutes

**Servings**: 2

**Ingredients**

- oz. almond flour
- ½ tsp ground cumin
- ½ tsp ground coriander
- oz. grated mozzarella cheese
- 4 oz. coconut milk, unsweetened
- Seasoning:
- ¼ tsp salt

- 2 tsp avocado oil

## Directions:

1. Take a medium bowl, place all the ingredients in it except for oil, and stir until well combined and smooth batter comes together.

2. Take a medium skillet pan, place it over medium heat, add 1 tsp oil and when hot, pour in half of the prepared batter, spread it evenly in a circular shape, then switch heat to the low level and cook for 2 minutes per side until golden brown and cooked.

3. Transfer dosa to a plate, then repeat with the remaining batter and serve.

**Nutrition**: 181 Calories; 16.5 g Fats; 6 g Protein; 2 g Net Carb; 0 g Fiber;

# Garlic Cheese Balls

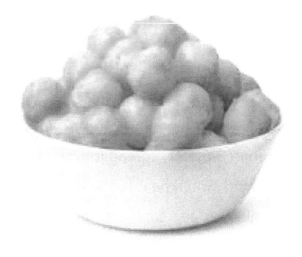

**Preparation Time**: 10 minutes

**Cooking Time**: 0 minutes

**Servings**: 2

## Ingredients

- 2 bacon sliced, cooked, chopped
- ½ tsp minced garlic
- 2 oz. cream cheese, softened
- 2 tbsp. sour cream
- 3 tbsp. grated parmesan cheese
- Seasoning:
- ½ tsp Italian seasoning

## Directions:

1. Take a medium bowl, place cheese in it, then add remaining ingredients except for bacon and stir until mixed.
2. Cover the bowl, let it refrigerate for 1 hour until chilled, and then shape the mixture into four balls.
3. Roll the balls in chopped bacon until coated, refrigerate for 30 minutes until firm, and then serve.

**Nutrition**: 335 Calories; 28.7 g Fats; 12.4 g Protein; 5.8 g Net Carb; 0 g Fiber;

# Cheddar and Green Onion Biscuits

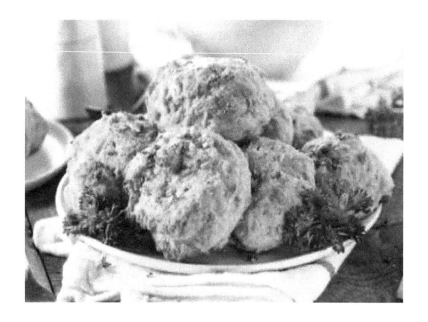

**Preparation Time**: 5 minutes;

**Cooking Time**: 8 minutes

**Servings**: 2

**Ingredients**

- 1 tsp chopped green onion
- 2 ½ tbsp. coconut flour
- 2 ½ tbsp. melted butter, unsalted
- 2 oz. grated cheddar cheese
- 1 egg
- Seasoning:

- 1/8 tsp baking powder
- ½ tsp garlic powder
- ¼ tsp salt
- 1/8 tsp ground black pepper

## Directions:

1. Turn on the oven, then set it to 400 degrees F and let it preheat.
2. Take a medium bowl, place flour in it, and then stir in garlic powder, baking powder, salt, and black pepper.
3. Take a separate medium bowl, crack the egg in it, whisk in butter until blended, and then whisk this mixture into the flour until incorporated and smooth.
4. Fold in green onion and cheese, then drop the mixture in the form of mounds onto a cookie sheet greased with oil and bake for 8 minutes until lightly browned.
5. When done, brush biscuit with some more melted butter and then serve.

**Nutrition**: 272 Calories; 23 g Fats; 11.5 g Protein; 4.5 g Net Carb; 0.7 g Fiber;

# Basil Wrapped Cheese Balls

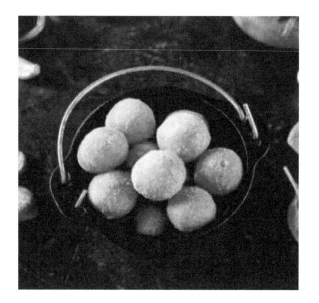

**Preparation Time**: 10 minutes

**Cooking Time**: 0 minutes

**Servings**: 2

**Ingredients**

- 2 oz. grated cheddar cheese
- 3 oz. grated mozzarella cheese
- 3 oz. grated parmesan cheese
- ¼ tsp ground black pepper
- 8 basil leaves

**Directions:**

1. Take a medium bowl, place all the cheeses in it, add black pepper, stir until blended, then cover the bowl and let it refrigerate for 30 minutes until firm.

2. Then shape the mixture into 1-inch long eight balls, then place each ball on the wide end of a basil leaf and roll it up.

3. Serve immediately.

**Nutrition**: 428 Calories; 31.4 g Fats; 28.9 g Protein; 7.5 g Net Carb; 0 g Fiber;

# Double Cheese Chips

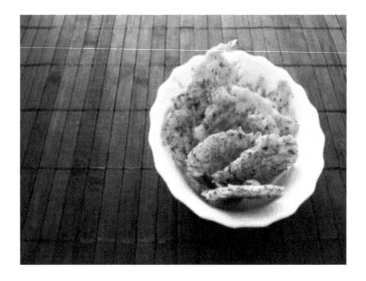

**Preparation Time**: 10 minutes;

**Cooking Time**: 10 minutes

**Servings**: 2

**Ingredients**

- 3 oz. grated cheddar cheese
- 5 oz. grated parmesan cheese
- 1/8 tsp onion powder
- 1/8 tsp ground cumin
- 1/8 tsp red chili powder
- Seasoning:
- 1/8 tsp salt

## Directions:

1. Turn on the oven, then set it to 400 degrees F and let it preheat.
2. Take a medium bowl, place cheeses in it, add salt, onion powder, cumin, and red chili powder and stir until mixed.
3. Take a baking pan, line it with parchment paper, spread cheese mixture on it in an even layer, and then bake for 10 minutes until cheese has melted and begin to crisp.
4. When done, remove the baking pan from the oven, let it cool completely and then cut it into triangles.
5. Serve.

**Nutrition**: 468 Calories; 34.2 g Fats; 30.3 g Protein; 9.3 g Net Carb; 0 g Fiber;

# Bacon Caprese with Parmesan

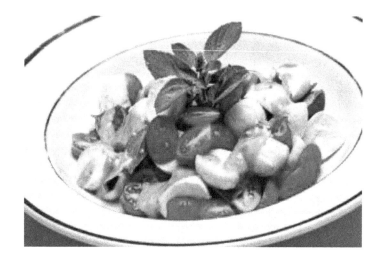

**Preparation Time**: 5 minutes

**Cooking Time**: 8 minutes

**Servings**: 2

## Ingredients

- 2 slices of bacon
- 2 Roma tomato, sliced
- 1 tsp balsamic vinegar
- 2 tbsp. avocado oil
- 1 tbsp. grated parmesan cheese
- Seasoning:

- ½ tsp salt
- ½ tsp ground black pepper

## Directions:

1. Take a frying pan, place it over medium heat and when hot, add bacon and cook for 3 to 4 minutes until crispy.
2. Transfer bacon to a cutting board, let it cool for 5 minutes and then chop it.
3. Turn on the broiler and let it preheat.
4. Take a medium baking sheet, line it with aluminum foil, spray with oil, spread tomato slices on it, and then drizzle with vinegar and oil.
5. Season with salt and black pepper, sprinkle with cheese and bacon and then broil tomatoes for 1 to 2 minutes until cheese has melted.
6. Serve.

**Nutrition**: 355 Calories; 28 g Fats; 18.6 g Protein; 5.7 g Net Carb; 2.3 g Fiber;

# Egg McMuffin Sandwich with Avocado and Bacon

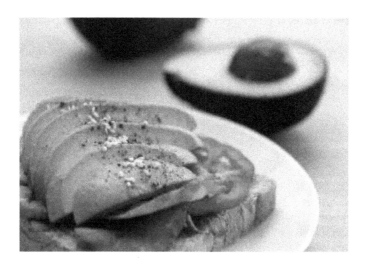

**Preparation Time**: 10 minutes

**Cooking Time**: 15 minutes

**Servings**: 2

**Ingredients**

- 2 eggs, yolks and egg whites separated
- 1/3 cup grated parmesan cheese
- 2 oz. cream cheese, softened
- 2 slices of bacon
- ½ of avocado, sliced
- Seasoning:

- 2/3 tsp salt
- 1 tsp avocado oil

## Directions:

1. Take a medium bowl, place egg yolks in it, add cream cheese, parmesan, and salt and whisk by using an electric blender until smooth.
2. Take another medium bowl, add egg whites, beat until stiff peaks form and then fold egg whites into egg yolk mixture until combined.
3. Take a skillet pan, place it over medium heat, add oil and when hot, add one-fourth of the batter, spread it into a 1-inch thick pancake, and then fry got 2 minutes per side until golden brown.
4. When done, let sandwiches cool for 5 minutes, top two muffins with bacon and avocado slices, cover the top with another muffin, and then serve as desired.

**Nutrition**: 355 Calories; 28 g Fats; 18.6 g Protein; 5.7 g Net Carb; 2.3 g Fiber;

# Hot Red Chili and Garlic Chutney

**Preparation Time**:  25 minutes

**Cooking Time:** 15 minutes

**Servings** 1

**Ingredients:**

- Red chilies, dried – 14
- Minced garlic – 5 teaspoons
- Salt – 1/8 teaspoon
- Water – 1 and ¼ cups

**Directions:**

1. Place chilies in a bowl, pour in water and let rest for 20 minutes.
2. Then drain red chilies, chop them and add to a blender.
3. Add remaining ingredients into the blender and pulse for 1 to 2 minutes until smooth.
4. Tip the sauce into a bowl and serve straight away.

**Nutrition:** calories: 100, fat: 1, fiber: 2, carbs: 6, protein: 7

# Red Chilies and Onion Chutney

**Preparation Time**: 15 minutes

**Cooking Time:** 15 minutes

**Servings** 2

**Ingredients:**

- Medium white onion, peeled and chopped – 1
- Minced garlic – 1 teaspoon
- Red chilies, chopped – 2
- Salt – ¼ teaspoon
- Sweet paprika – 1 teaspoon
- Avocado oil – 2 teaspoons
- Water – ¼ cup

**Directions:**

1. Place a medium skillet pan over medium-high heat, add oil and when hot, add onion, garlic, and chilies.
2. Cook onions for 5 minutes or until softened, then season with salt and paprika and pour in water.
3. Stir well and cook for 5 minutes.
4. Then spoon the chutney into a bowl and serve.

**Nutrition:** calories: 121, fat: 2, fiber: 6, carbs: 9,

protein: 5

# Fast Guacamole

**Preparation Time**: 10 minutes

**Cooking Time:** 15 minutes

**Servings** 12

**Ingredients:**

- Medium avocados, peeled, pitted and cubed – 3
- Medium tomato, cubed – 1
- Chopped cilantro – ¼ cup
- Medium red onion, peeled and chopped – 1
- Salt – ½ teaspoon
- Ground white pepper – ¼ teaspoon
- Lime juice – 3 tablespoons

**Directions:**

1. Place all the ingredients for the salad in a medium bowl and stir until combined.
2. Serve guacamole straightaway as an appetizer.

**Nutrition:** calories: 87, fat: 4, fiber: 4, carbs: 8, protein: 2

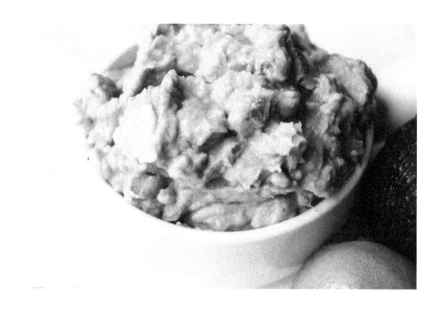

# Coconut Dill Dip

**Preparation Time**: 10 minutes

**Cooking Time:** 15 minutes

**Servings** 10

**Ingredients:**

- Chopped white onion – 1 tablespoon
- Parsley flakes – 2 teaspoons
- Chopped dill – 2 teaspoons
- Salt – ¼ teaspoon
- Coconut cream – 1 cup
- Avocado mayonnaise – ½ cup

**Directions:**

1. Place all the ingredients for the dip in a medium bowl and whisk until combined.
2. Serve the dip with vegetable sticks as a side dish.

**Nutrition:** calories: 102, fat: 3, fiber: 1, carbs: 2, protein: 2

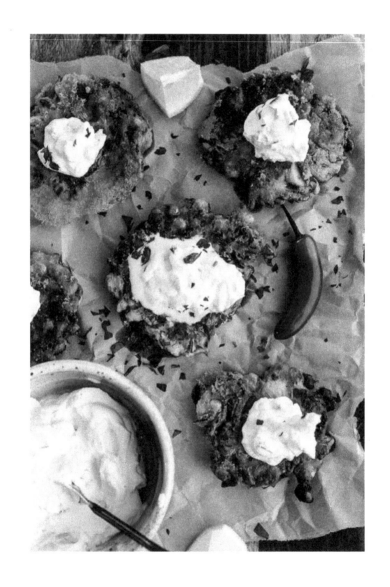

# Creamy Mango and Mint Dip

**Preparation Time**: 10 minutes

**Cooking Time:** 15 minutes

**Servings** 4

**Ingredients:**

- Medium green chili, chopped – 1
- Medium white onion, peeled and chopped – 1
- Grated ginger – 1 tablespoon
- Minced garlic – 1 teaspoon
- Salt – 1/8 teaspoon
- Ground black pepper – 1/8 teaspoon
- Cumin powder – 1 teaspoon
- Mango powder – 1 teaspoon
- Mint leaves – 2 cups
- Coriander leaves – 1 cup
- Cashew yogurt – 4 tablespoons

**Directions:**

1. Place all the ingredients for the dip in a blender and pulse for 1 to 2 minutes or until smooth.
2. Tip the dip into small cups and serve straightaway.

**Nutrition**: calories: 100, fat: 2, fiber: 3, carbs: 7, protein: 5

# Creamy Crab Dip

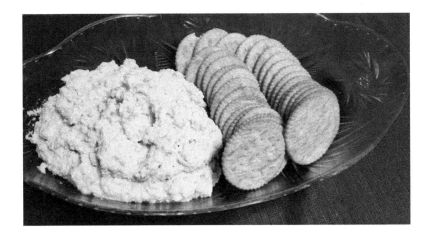

**Preparation Time** 5 minutes

**Cooking Time:** 10 minutes

**Servings** 12

**Ingredients:**

- Crab meat, chopped – 1 pound
- Chopped white onion – 2 tablespoons
- Minced garlic – 1 tablespoon
- Lemon juice – 2 tablespoons
- Cream cheese, cubed – 16 ounces
- Avocado mayonnaise – 1/3 cup
- Grape juice – 2 tablespoons

**Directions:**

1. Place all the ingredients for the dip in a medium bowl and stir until combined.

2. Divide dip evenly between small bowls and serve as a party dip.

**Nutrition:** Calories: 100, Fat: 4, Fiber: 1, Carbs: 4, Protein: 4

# Creamy Cheddar and Bacon Spread with Almonds

**Preparation Time**:  10 minutes

**Cooking Time:** 10 minutes

**Servings** 12

**Ingredients:**

- Bacon, cooked and chopped – 12 ounces
- Chopped sweet red pepper – 2 tablespoons
- Medium white onion, peeled and chopped – 1
- Salt – ¾ teaspoon
- Ground black pepper – ½ teaspoon
- Almonds, chopped – ½ cup
- Cheddar cheese, grated – 1 pound
- Avocado mayonnaise – 2 cups

**Directions:**

1. Place all the ingredients for the dip in a medium bowl and stir until combined.
2. Divide dip evenly between small bowls and serve as a party dip.

**Nutrition:** calories: 184, fat: 12, fiber: 1, carbs: 4, protein: 5

# Green Tabasco Devilled Eggs

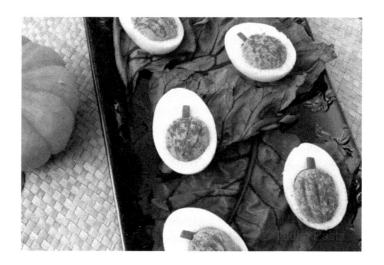

**Preparation Time**: 20 minutes

**Cooking Time:** 10 minutes

**Servings**: 6

**Ingredients:**

- 6 Eggs
- 1/3 cup Mayonnaise
- 1 ½ tbsp. Green Tabasco
- Salt and Pepper, to taste

**Directions:**

1. Place the eggs in a saucepan over medium heat and pour boiling water over, enough to cover them.
2. Cook for 6-8 minutes.
3. Place in an ice bath to cool.
4. When safe to handle, peel the eggs and slice them in half.
5. Scoop out the yolks and place in a bowl.
6. Add the remaining ingredients.
7. Whisk to combine.
8. Fill the egg holes with the mixture.
9. Serve and enjoy!

**Nutrition:** Calories 175 Total Fats 17g Net Carbs: 5g Protein 6g Fiber: 1g

# Herbed Cheese Balls

**Preparation Time**: 30 MIN

**Cooking Time:** 10 minutes

**Servings**: 20

**Ingredients:**

- 1/3 cup grated Parmesan Cheese
- 3 tbsp. Heavy Cream
- 4 tbsp. Butter, melted
- ¼ tsp Pepper
- 2 Eggs
- 1 cup Almond Flour
- ¼ cup Basil Leaves
- ¼ cup Parsley Leaves
- 2 tbsp. chopped Cilantro Leaves
- 1/3 cup crumbled Feta Cheese

**Directions:**

1. Place the ingredients in your food processor.
2. Pulse until the mixture becomes smooth.
3. Transfer to a bowl and freeze for 20 minutes or so, to set.
4. Shale the mixture into 20 balls.

5. Meanwhile, preheat the oven to 350 degrees F.

6. Arrange the cheese balls on a lined baking sheet.

7. Place in the oven and bake for 10 minutes.

8. Serve and enjoy!

**Nutrition:** Calories 60 Total Fats 5g Net Carbs: 8g Protein 2g Fiber: 1g

# Cheesy Salami Snack

**Preparation Time**: 30 MIN

**Cooking Time:** 10 minutes

**Servings**: 6

**Ingredients:**

- 4 ounces Cream Cheese
- 7 ounces dried Salami
- ¼ cup chopped Parsley

**Directions:**

1. Preheat the oven to 325 degrees F.
2. Slice the salami thinly (I got 30 slices).
3. Arrange the salami on a lined sheet and bake for 15 minutes.
4. Arrange on a serving platter and top each salami slice with a bit of cream cheese.
5. Serve and enjoy!

**Nutrition:** Calories 139 Total Fats 15g Net Carbs: 1g Protein 9g Fiber: 0g

# Pesto & Olive Fat Bombs

**Preparation Time**: 25 MIN

**Cooking Time:** 10 minutes

**Servings**: 8

**Ingredients:**

- 1 cup Cream Cheese
- 10 Olives, sliced
- 2 tbsp. Pesto Sauce
- ½ cup grated Parmesan Cheese

**Directions:**

1. Place all of the ingredients in a bowl.
2. Stir well to combine.
3. Place in the freezer and freeze for 15-20 minutes, to set.
4. Shape into 8 balls.
5. Serve and enjoy!

**Nutrition:** Calories 123 Total Fats 13g Net Carbs: 3g Protein 4g Fiber: 3g

# Cheesy Broccoli Nuggets

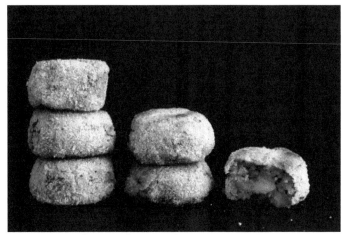

**Preparation Time**: 25 MIN

**Cooking Time:** 10 minutes

**Servings**: 4

**Ingredients:**

- 1 cup shredded Cheese
- ¼ cup Almond Flour
- 2 cups Broccoli Florets, steamed in the microwave for 5 minutes
- 2 Egg Whites
- Salt and Pepper, to taste

**Directions:**

1. Preheat the oven to 350 degrees F.

2. Place the broccoli florets in a bowl and mash them with a potato masher.

3. Add the remaining ingredients and mix well with your hands, until combined.

4. Line a baking sheet with parchment paper.

5. Drop 20 scoops of the mixture onto the sheet.

6. Place in the oven and bake for 20 minutes or until golden.

7. Serve and enjoy!

**Nutrition:** Calories 145 Total Fats 9g Net Carbs: 4g Protein 10g Fiber: 1g

# Salmon Fat Bombs

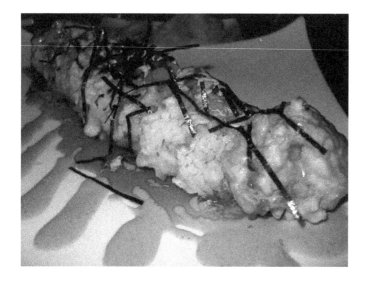

**Preparation Time**: 90 MIN

**Cooking Time:** 50 minutes

**Servings**: 6

**Ingredients:**

- ½ cup Cream Cheese
- 1 ½ tbsp. chopped Dill
- 1 ¾ ounces Smoked Salmon, sliced
- 1 tbsp. Lemon Juice
- 1/3 cup Butter
- ¼ tsp Red Pepper Flakes
- ¼ tsp Garlic Powder

- Pinch of Salt
- ¼ tsp Pepper

## Directions:

1. Place the butter, salmon, lemon juice, and cream cheese, in your food processor.
2. Add the seasonings.
3. Pulse until smooth.
4. Drop spoonfuls of the mixture onto a lined dish.
5. Sprinkle with the dill.
6. Place in the fridge for about 80 minutes.
7. Serve and enjoy!

**Nutrition:** Calories 145 Total Fats 16g Net Carbs: 7g Protein 3g Fiber: 1g

# Guacamole Bacon Bombs

**Preparation Time**: 30 MIN

**Cooking Time:** 10 minutes

**Servings**: 6

**Ingredients:**

- 1 tsp minced Garlic
- ¼ cup Butter
- ½ Avocado, flesh scooped out
- 1 tbsp. Lime Juice
- 1 tbsp. chopped Cilantro
- 4 Bacon Slices, cooked and crumbled
- 3 tbsp. diced Shallots
- Salt and Pepper, to taste
- 1 tbsp. minced Jalapeno

**Directions:**

1. Place all of the ingredients, except the bacon, in your food processor.
2. Pulse until smooth. Alternatively, you can do this by whisking in a bowl. Just keep in mind that this way you will have chunks of garlic and jalapenos.
3. Transfer to a bowl and place in the freezer.

4. Freeze for 20 minutes, or until set.

5. Shape into 6 balls.

6. Coat them with bacon pieces.

7. Serve and enjoy!

**Nutrition:** Calories 155 Total Fats 15g Net Carbs: 4g Protein 4g Fiber: 3g

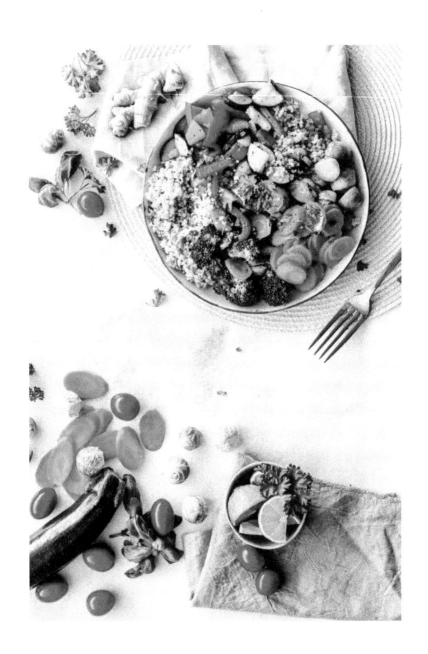

# CONCLUSION

The things to watch out for when coming off keto are weight gain, bloating, more energy, and feeling hungry. The weight gain is nothing to freak out over; perhaps, you might not even gain any. It all depends on your diet, how your body processes carbs, and, of course, water weight. The length of your keto diet is a significant factor in how much weight you have lost, which is caused by the reduction of carbs. The bloating will occur because of the reintroduction of fibrous foods and your body getting used to digesting them again. The bloating van lasts for a few days to a few weeks. You will feel like you have more energy because carbs break down into glucose, which is the body's primary source of fuel. You may also notice better brain function and the ability to work out more.

Whether you have met your weight loss goals, your life changes, or you simply want to eat whatever you want again. You cannot just suddenly start consuming carbs again for it will shock your system. Have an idea of what you want to allow back into your consumption slowly. Be familiar with portion sizes and stick to that amount of carbs for the first few times you eat post-keto.

Start with non-processed carbs like whole grain, beans, and fruits. Start slow and see how your body responds before resolving to add carbs one meal at a time.

The ketogenic diet is the ultimate tool you can use to plan your future. Can you picture being more involved, more productive and efficient, and more relaxed and energetic? That future is possible for you, and it does not have to be a complicated process to achieve that vision. You can choose right now to be healthier and slimmer and more fulfilled tomorrow. It is possible with the ketogenic diet.

It does not just improve your physical health but your mental and emotional health as well. This diet improves your health holistically. Do not give up now as there will be quite a few days where you may think to yourself, "Why am I doing this?" and to answer that, simply focus on the goals you wish to achieve.

A good diet enriched with all the proper nutrients is our best shot of achieving an active metabolism and efficient lifestyle. A lot of people think that the Keto diet is simply for people who are interested in losing weight. You will find that it is quite the opposite. There are intense keto diets where only 5 percent of the diet comes from carbs, 20 percent is from protein, and 75 percent is from fat. But even a modified version of this which involves consciously choosing foods low in carbohydrate and high in healthy fats is good enough.

Thanks for reading this book. I hope it has provided you with enough insight to get you going. Don't put off getting started. The sooner you begin this diet, the sooner you'll start to notice an improvement in your health and well-being.

CPSIA information can be obtained
at www.ICGtesting.com
Printed in the USA
BVHW052028120421
604747BV00005B/313